Essential Oils for Winter

Natural Healing and Wellbeing

Table of Contents

Introduction: Wintertime Aroma!

Winter can be a beautiful time of year, and the snow covered trees may seem inviting, but the significant drop in temperature, and prolonged exposure to the harsh elements, can really wreak some havoc on your skin, hair, nails, immune system, and general well being! Like many, I get dry and cracked skin just about every winter, and am usually looking for a good lotion in order to combat the dryness. In this book we will go over just such a solution.

Finding you the best essential oil to handle any problem you might have during the winter season. And speaking of the winter season, besides the beautiful sights and sounds of the yuletide, there is also one other sense that is quite often invoked during this magical time of year; the sense of smell. Smell has become quite a part of the winter season; we like to smell our pumpkin spice coffee, as well as our pumpkin pie.

There is also often a hint of Frankincense and Myrrh in the air during the winter months, and who can forget the fresh scent of winter pine trees? The point is, the winter is full of some very special essential oils; you just have to know how to use them. And that is precisely what this book is for. Read further so that you can learn exactly what essential oils you should have on stock this winter and what purpose they might serve you during the colder months of the year.

Chapter 1: Wintertime Essential Oils to Boost Your Immune System

The winter is a really fun time of year, but it can really wear out your immune system. Cold weather automatically sends our immune defenses into a downward spiral, but there are some ways that you can enhance and even boost your immune system with the use of just a few simple essential oils. Read this chapter to find out more!

Frankincense Oil

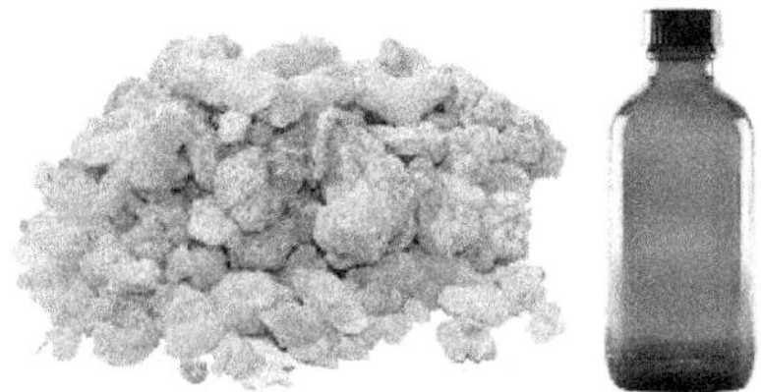

Because of a few Magi, gifts of Frankincense and Myrrh are in quite a bit of demand during the winter months. But it is Frankincense that works the best when it comes to boosting the immune system. This essential oil is able to cleanse the whole body of those who apply it, killing germs upon contact. If you are at all feeling under the weather this winter, or even afraid that you might be, you should really give Frankincense a try.

Along with boosting the immune system, Frankincense has also been discovered to fight cancer. And its unique ability to cross the blood brain barrier, makes it especially important when boosting the immune systems ability to battle cancers of the brain. One of the best ways to administer frankincense oil is to simply massage a couple drops right into your hands and feet.

Your body will quickly absorb this frankincense through your extremities and circulate its properties throughout your body. On cold winter mornings just massage in a little bit of this oil, and you will have a valuable immune system booster to help you brave the harsh elements. Frankincense oil also works well when it is burned as incense, but no matter how you use it, this oil is going give you that boost that you need.

Tea Tree Oil

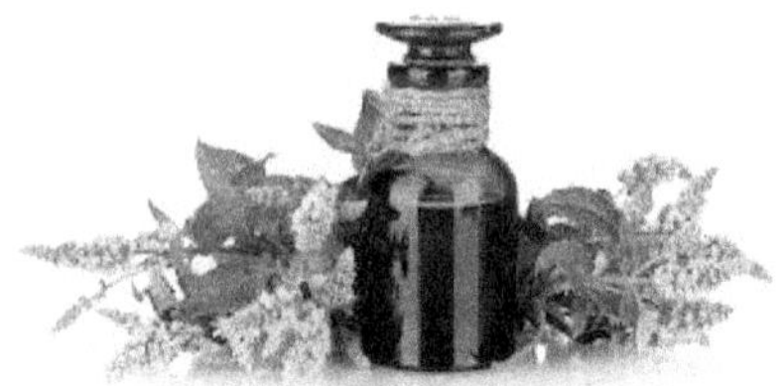

This oil is often burned in the house as incense during the course of the winter months. It works as a great disinfectant and just by breathing the aroma of this oil, you can get a significant boost in your immune system. This oil is very holistic in nature and can work to take care of your general immune health and well being. Most importantly tea tree oil plays a vital role in enhancing white blood cell production. Use this special blend of tea tree oil in order to boost your immune system this winter!

Eucalyptus Oil

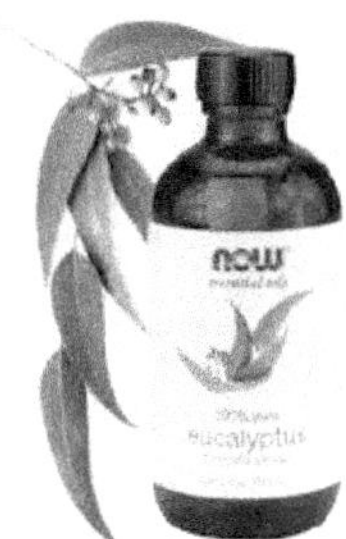

This essential oil when rubbed in the skin or breathed in the air can serve to give your immune system a much needed restart. Eucalyptus oil has very powerful antibacterial and antiviral properties that serve to bolster immune health. This same eucalyptus oil then goes on to enhance oxygen production in cell tissue, allowing our bodies to heal themselves much faster at a cellular level. Eucalyptus oil is also magnificent at reducing fevers.

So if you are feeling a bit feverish this winter, a cold compress with eucalyptus oil would do you well to reduce that troubling bout of fever. Eucalyptus has been used to treat everything from the flu to strep throat during the harsh winter months. It would be a good idea to stock up on this powerful agent during the wintertime. The best way to use eucalyptus is to breathe in the aroma through incense or through direct inhalation from an essential oil container. Be sure to give eucalyptus oil a try this winter, your immune system will thank you for it later!

Ginger Oil

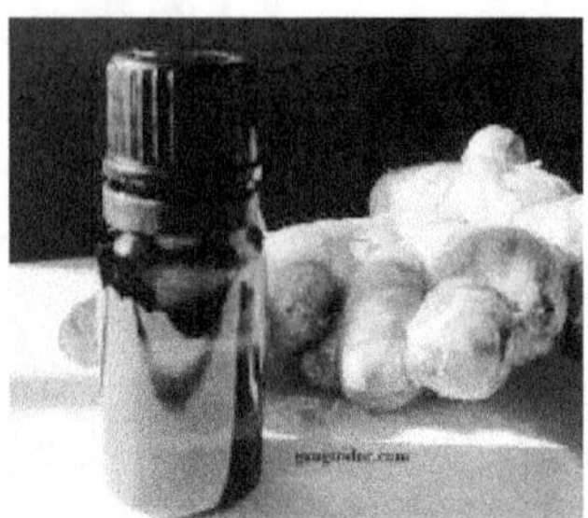

Ginger is a wonderful anti inflammatory agent, and takes on a significant role when it comes to immune health. If you feel that your immune system is weakening during the cold and flu season of the long winter months you might want to give ginger oil a try. Regular doses of ginger help to regulate your blood pressure, and since a stable blood pressure is something on which your immune system's health depends, you should make sure that you keep a batch of ginger around during the winter time. Just expose yourself to this oil either through direct application or through aromatherapy and you will reap the benefit of a greatly enhanced immune system.

Oregano Oil

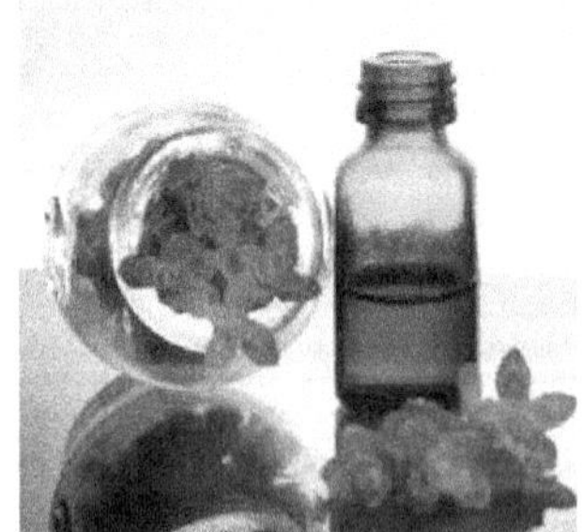

The name "oregano" actually comes from the Greek words "oros" and "ganos" which mean "mountain and "joy" respectively Making the name Oregano translate into something like, "Joy of the Mountain". This essential oil works to shield the immune system from dangerous free radicals that accumulate in our cells. A steady routine of this oil can help cleanse your body of these elements that can be so harmful to the immune system.

During the wintertime you should make sure you have a healthy batch of oregano around to keep your immune system nice and strong. In order to use this essential oil you should simply rub it on like you would perfume, just putting a small dab on your neck and chest so that you can reap the benefits of this essential oil's aroma all throughout your day. You might end up smelling like a walking plate of pasta, but if it means giving your immune system a much deserved boost this winter, you should give it a try!

Saffron Oil

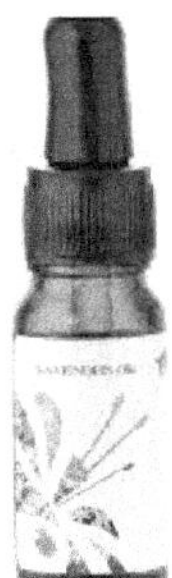

A serious immune booster, Saffron oil is known for its ability to fight sluggishness and depression during the winter months. Just put a little bit of this oil on your skin and massage it in, and see the difference in your immune health! The oil is derived from the stem of the Saffron plant. Extracted in its purest form it just takes a few drops of this oil massaged into the skin in order to see a difference in immune health. As soon as your body absorbs the proactive immune benefits of this oil you will be in great shape all winter long. Never take the powerful components of this oil for granted, if you are feeling a bit under the weather during the cold winter months, just give saffron oil a try!

Astragalus Oil

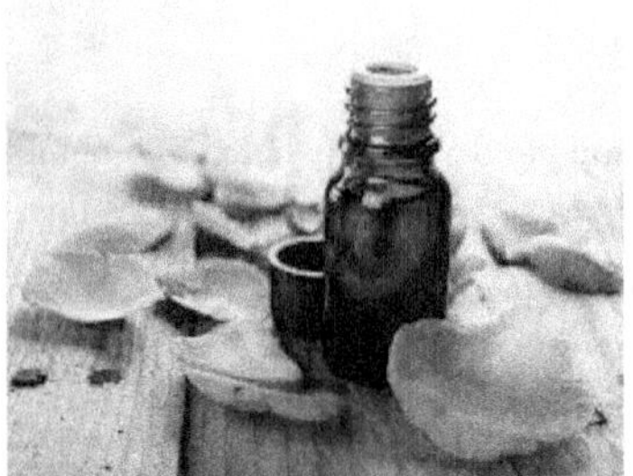

This oil has been used in Chinese medicine for thousands of years as a natural enhancement to the immune system. During the winter months when the cold and flu system are in high gear, it would be wise for you to have some of this essential oil on hand. This essential oil works best rubbed into the outer epidermis layers. But this essential oil is potent so just make sure that you dilute it well, with a carrier oil base in order to distribute it to the skin. Once your oil is diluted like this you can then apply it liberally to neck and chest, helping to bolster your immunity from sickness during the winter.

Echinacea Oil

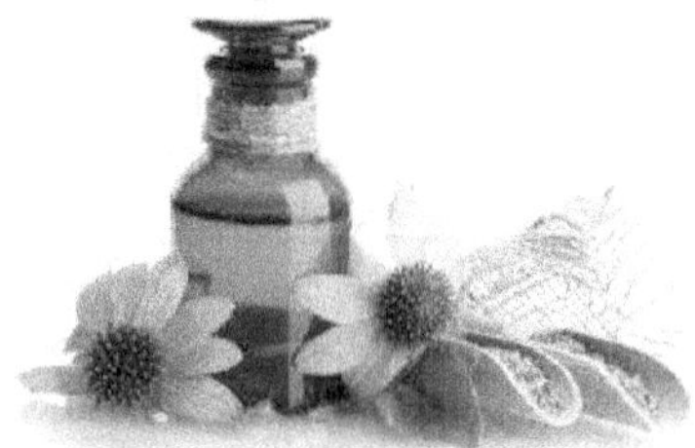

This oil actually works well as both an antiviral and an antibiotic. Echinacea oil strengthens the immune system on two levels, it serves to cleanse the body of contaminates and it also keeps down inflammation; two very important aspects of immune health. Native Americans who lived in the northern plains of the United States often used Echinacea as an important supplement during the winter for this vey same important reason. So don't just take my word for it, take the word of countless generations of Native Americans that have used it to treat illness. This essential oil kills germs on contact so be sure to rub it into your palms fairly regularly during the winter season.

Chapter 2: Essential Oil for Memory and Mental Focus

The winter can really dull our senses and sometimes we could all use a little boost. Essential oil is just the boost that we need to reestablish that mental focus and enrich our faltering memory. In this chapter learn about some of the best essential oil compounds that can truly make you have some good memories this winter!

Coriander Oil

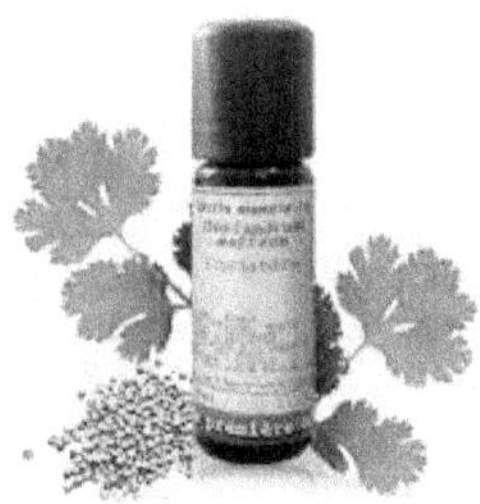

This essential oil has an amazing ability when it comes to stimulating blood flow in the brain, and as a result greatly benefits memory and concentration. It also helps the body relax, and with this relaxation comes enhanced mental focus. Coriander is also known as a natural "chelator", an agent that can remove toxic metals, such as cadmum, aluminum, mercury, and even lead from tissue.

These toxic materials are known to be great disrupters when it comes to mental focus, the more that can be naturally removed through the application of coriander oil to the skin the better off you will be. So if you feel like your memory and focus this winter are starting to slip, get yourself a grip by getting a heart dose of coriander oil this winter!

Grapefruit Oil

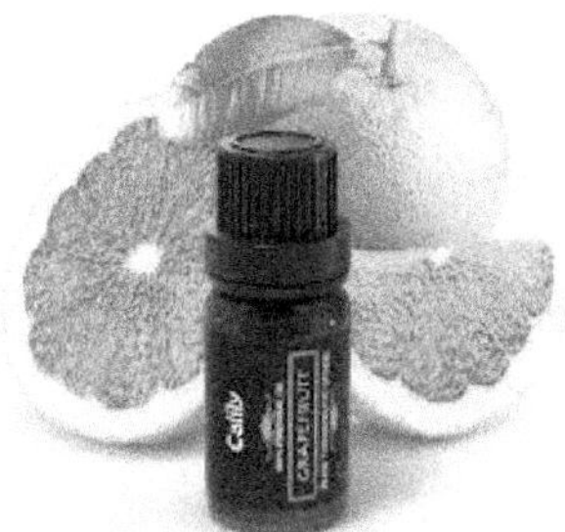

The oil of this tasty fruit can enrich your very brain cells, pumping extra blood in your vessels and brining more oxygen to your brain. The antimicrobial properties of this essential oil also serve to cleanse the skin, keeping dangerous contaminants from affecting your cognitive function. The most prevalent material of grapefruit oil is a substance called "limonene" which makes up about 95% of the oil itself.

The power of grapefruit essential oil should never be underestimated and can be used to eliminate salmonella and even e coli. Grapefruit oil also has important antifungal properties that can help prevent diseases of the brain such as meningitis. This essential oil is a powerful agent for wellness. For health, memory, and mental focus during the winter months, you should give grapefruit oil a try.

Rose Oil

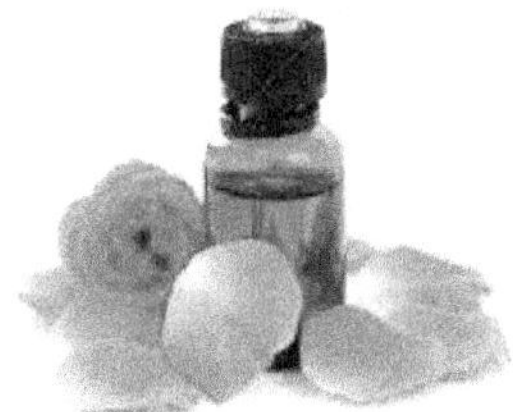

Rose oil gives a definite boost in memory and mental focus. In fact, a recent scientific study has found that the sniffing of rosemary essential oil can improve memory by as much as 75%. If you feel that you are getting a bit forgetful over the course of the winter just inhale a good batch of rose oil and much of your winter brain fog will dissipate. Rose oil will work to clear out any interference in your mind and enhance the stimulation of your cognitive function. In order to stay sharp and focused this winter you should give rose essential oil a try.

Neroli Oil

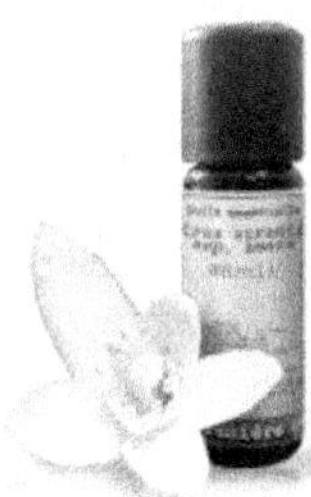

Neroli has an amazing way of restoring mental focus and boosting memory. This essential oil is also very relaxing, and this goes hand in hand with bringing about a relaxed cognitive function to the brain. Just rub some of this essential oil into your skin and you will soon start to see a noticeable difference in your overall memory and mental focus. This neroli oil will give you mental clarity all winter long.

Jasmine Oil

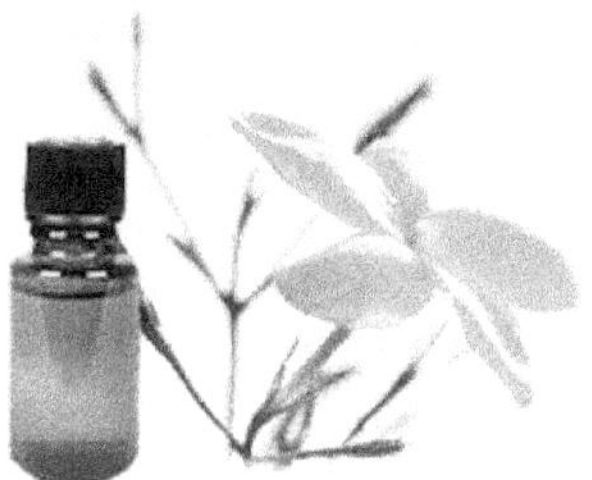

Jasmine smells great, and its aroma can also make you remember stuff! The aroma of jasmine has been known to enhance mental clarity, focus, and even libido! The best way to apply jasmine is by diluting it in a good carrier oil base and then applying it directly to the skin in either a compress or an aromatic massage! This essential oil can do you wonders during the harsh winter months, so it wouldn't be a bad idea to keep a large supply on hand. So if you are feeling like you are in a bit of a mental funk this winter, just give some jasmine essential oil a try!

Cyprus Oil

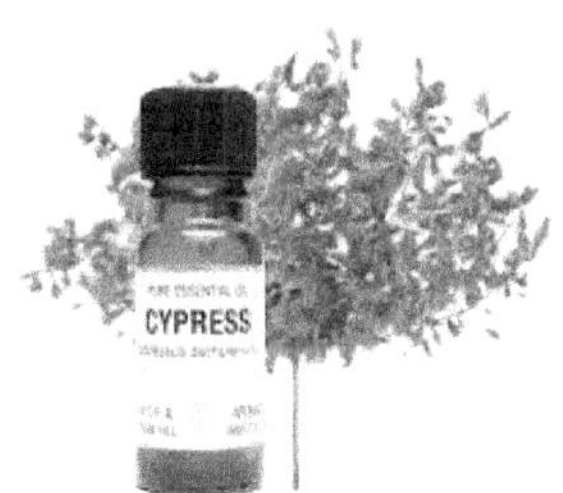

During the winter months the evergreen aroma of Cyprus is a pleasing addition to the season. Just a few drops of this oil can greatly aid your overall memory and mental focus. Cyprus oil has even been shown effective in treating the symptoms of Alzheimer's and dementia. This oil can be administered through incense infused aromas or through direct application to the skin. Keep your memories crisp this winter season by using Cyprus oil!

Basil Oil

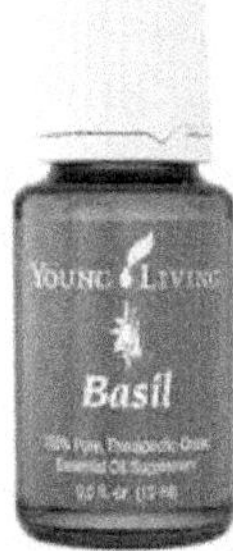

Just one good whiff of basil oil and you will feel invigorated with renewed mental focus. Basil oil has been especially effective for women going through menopause. This essential oil can bring back mental focus and hormone balance when taken on a routine basis. The best way to administer basil essential oil is to inhale it directly or burn it in your general vicinity as incense. In order to stay focused and on task this winter keep a good supply of basil essential oil.

Coconut Oil

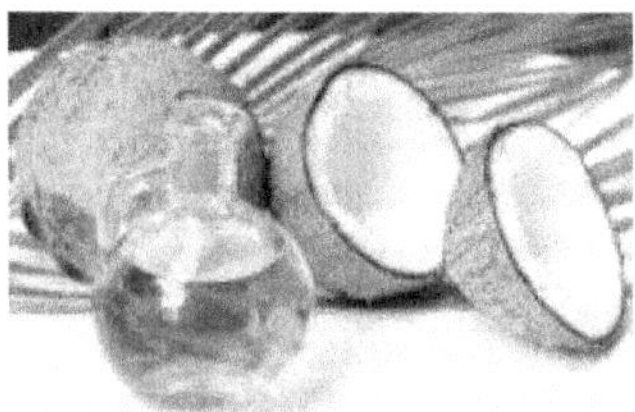

If you feel like your memory is on the decline, then you might want to give coconut essential oil a try. Coconut oil has been proven to aid memory, and has even been used to treat Alzheimer's. If you feel like your mind is being bogged down in a heavy fog this winter just try some coconut oil. The best means of application is direct, by rubbing this oil right into your skin. Don't hesitate to use coconut essential oil this winter!

Bergamot Oil

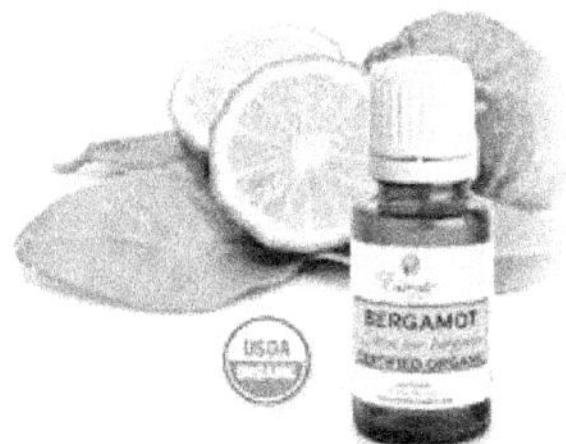

This oil can help to foster mental clarity in just about anyone who uses it. It also helps boost your memory. Just add a few drops of this oil to a humidifier and let it fill up the air in your home, and you will have all the memory and mental clarity you can handle this winter. The aroma of this oil will help you to improve your mood as well as improve your mental focus. So keep a hearty helping of bergamot essential oil in stock for when the blizzard hits!

Chapter 3: Essential Oils for Wintertime Cosmetic Health

The winter weather can really take a toll on our skin, making it dry and flaky, but if you have the right kind of essential oil you can combat all of these dreadful wintertime cosmetic deficits. Here in this chapter we have compiled and catalogued some of the best in essential oil based wintertime cosmetic health care!

Ylang Ylang Oil

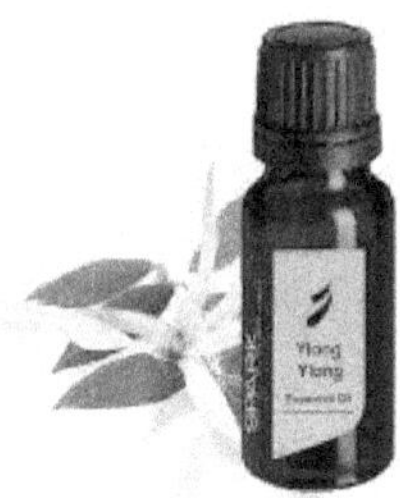

Ylang Ylang oil is actually really good for your skin and hair. Ylang ylang can do quite a bit to promote the production of sebum and eliminate dryness. Most scalp problems are a result of malfunctioning sebum glands in the scalp; ylang ylang stimulates these glands and boosts them back up to normal production levels. Ylang ylang also works well to regulate any hormone imbalances that may be present. This is great news for those of us that feel just a little bit off balance during the winter season. The change in weather can alter our body chemistry more than we realize, so keep your cupboards well stocked with this great essential oil during the winter.

Vetiver Oil

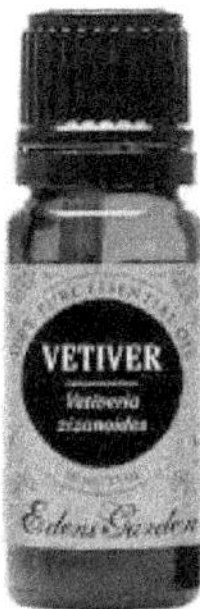

This essential oil is extracted from the roots of a special kind of grass that originates from India. It has been used for thousands of years to reduce dark blemishes and to create smoother, much more rejuvenated skin. Vetiver essential oil works as a great natural moisturizer, giving much needed moisture to dry skin, allowing it to heal itself from the replenishing nutrients that this oil provides. The result is a much more even complexion with a much more firm overall density in appearance.

When applied to the scalp, vetiver can also relax and coat hair follicles promoting growth and healing for damaged hair. My wife dyes her hair a lot, and as a result often has damaged hair. She used to use this very blend of essential oil however, and she had great results when it came to replenishing her damaged hair follicles. Whether you dye your hair or not however, the sheer cold of winter can do much the same damage to your hair, so consider using this essential oil to counterbalance this damage. This winter consider giving vetiver essential oil a try.

Patchouli Oil

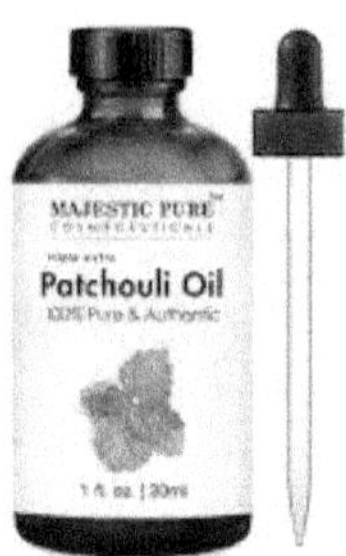

This funny looking plant with its puffy leaves can create much benefit for cosmetic beauty during the winter months. The essential oil extracted from this plant comes in an iconic amber brown, almost taking on the cadence of a good glass of beer. But this isn't a Budweiser! This is a skin and hair beautifier! This oil does well to treat problems of the scalp, as well as outer skin layer problems such as eczema, dermatitis, and dandruff.

Patchouli is a natural skin cell regenerator, and greatly hastens the healing of sores and cuts, and eventually, with regular treatment, even scars can be removed by the application of patchouli oil. Patchouli oil is a soothing agent for cracked skin and nourishes weak and brittle nails, all of which are common ailment of harsh winter weather. After so many months of going out in the ice and snow my hands can get pretty severely cracked and dry, but with a soothing agent like patchouli oil, dry cracked hands aren't a problem anymore! Don't forget to get your very own blend of patchouli oil this winter!

Lemon Oil

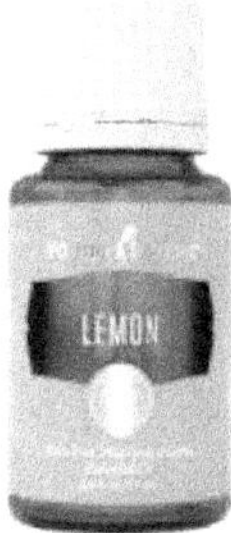

Lemon oil actually works well on oily scalps, and just a liberal lathering on the face can do much to exfoliate the skin and prevent pimples. Another cosmetic aspect of using lemon oil is as a hair lightener, this essential oil provides a natural way of lightening hair. Lemon essential oil has many important antiseptic, anti-inflammatory, and antibacterial elements that contribute to cosmetic health. One of the best ways to apply this oil to the skin is to simply place a few drops in your bathwater and allow the diluted oil to cleanse your skin while you bathe.

But if you would simply like to use this essential oil as a facial cleanser this can be easily done by putting just one drop on a cotton ball, before soaking the cotton ball with water, and then applying directly to the face. This sort of facial cleanser is highly effective when it comes to fighting acne. The reason why lemon oil is so effective I fighting acne is that it works as a natural astringent removing extra oil from the skin, and helping to minimize pores. Lemon oil also has quite a pleasant aroma and can be used as a cosmetic perfume. All of these benefits provide us with great reasons to keep lemon essential oil on the shelf this winter.

Thyme Oil

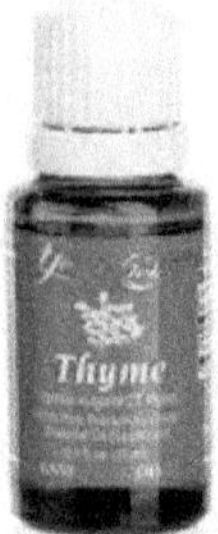

This essential oil works well to increase blood flow to the scalp, as well as providing a layer of protection against harmful microbes. Thyme is a great cleansing agent and works to remove harmful contaminants. Thyme is also good for oily skin, helping to relieve clogs in your pores while smoothing out your complexion. In order to keep your cosmetic health in great shape this winter give thyme essential oil a try.

Clary Sage Oil

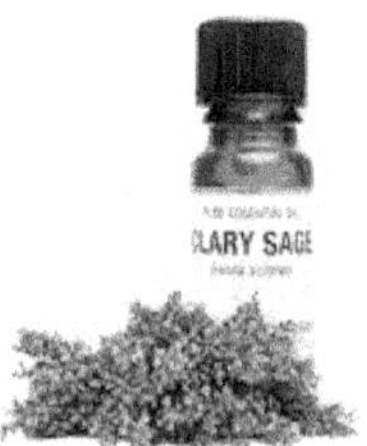

Clary Sage essential oil is extracted through steam distillation from the plant's leaves. This oil can actually do much to encourage hair growth and reverse the course of damaged hair follicles. If you have an oil scalp, rub this oil right into your hair and it will do much to soak up any excess oil. Clary Sage oil also works well as a facial cleanser, dilute a few drops with water and use it to wash your face during the harsh winter, so that you can have a clear and blemish free complexion. If you are in need of giving yourself a little cosmetic boost during the colder months of the year, you should keep a bottle of clary sage oil handy for just such an occasion.

Cedar Oil

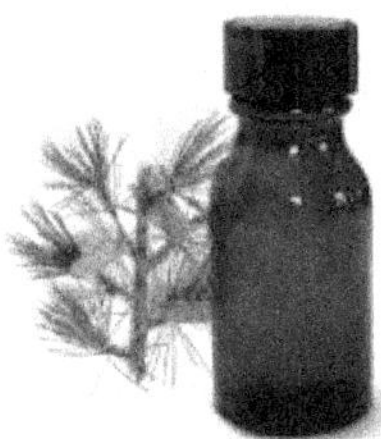

This oil eliminates dandruff, and replenishes depleted sebum oil deposits in the scalp getting rid of most symptoms of involved with having a dry scalp. This oil also provides much needed stimulation of hair follicles and blood circulation allowing for resurgence in hair growth. For best results just mix this oil right into your shampoo and apply it directly to your hair. Along with hair health, cedar essential oil can also do a lot for that cracked wintertime skin. The winter elements can make having smooth skin a tough prospect, but when you frequently lather your skin in cedar oil, it will be replenished in not time. Stock up on cedar oil for the winter!

Chamomile Oil

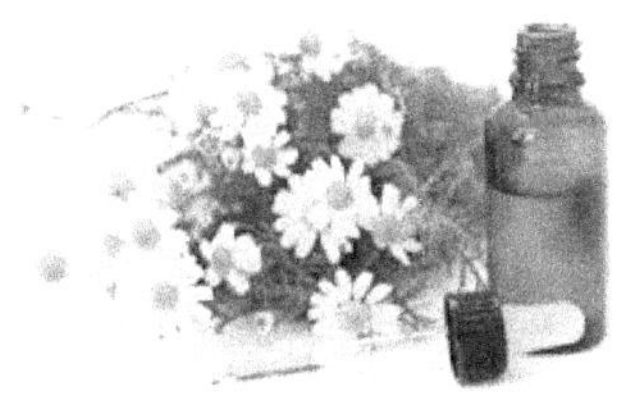

There is great potential in the anti-inflammatory power of chamomile oil. Rub this oil right into your scalp and it will eliminate any latent dandruff. This oil is a great anti-inflammatory agent, and as such, it works really well as a proactive agent against acne. This essential oil has been proven to keep skin clean and clear. Chamomile oil also works well to treat rashes and other skin irritations that are common during the winter months.

Rosemary Oil

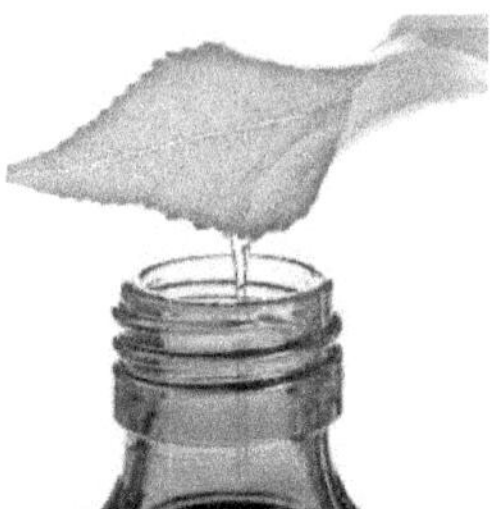

Rosemary oil is actually very efficient at slowing down the advent of graying hair. This oil can stimulate the roots of your hair, helping them t hang on to their original pigmentation. This oil also works as a great exfoliant on the skin. Rosemary also works as a great facial cleanser reducing the outbreak of acne and other skin surface difficulties. Regular doses or rosemary during the winter will give your face a healthy, glowing sheen. Make sure you keep some on hand during those long cold winters.

Lavender Oil

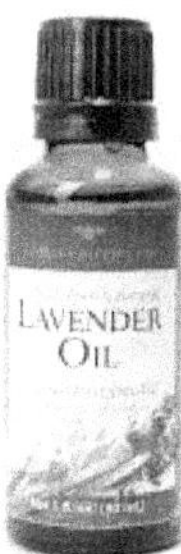

This oil provides much needed stimulation of the scalp and works to get rid of dandruff. This oil is also a great facial cleanser and exfoliant known to fight the spread of acne in those that apply it. Lavender also works well as a cleanser and facial toner. For those of us who have developed them, lavender oil can smooth out wrinkles, and greatly diminish many signs of the aging process. Many common problems that our skin suffers through during the winter months such as dryness and cracking, can be fixed with regular application of lavender oil to our skin.

Chapter 4: Essential oil for Energy and Metabolism

If you feel a little sluggish, and you find it hard to get out of bed on those cold winter mornings instead of reaching for that double shot espresso, reach for the essential oil! Because there are quite a few essential oil blends that can boost your energy while boosting your metabolism all at the same time. Here are a few of the best examples!

Fennel Oil

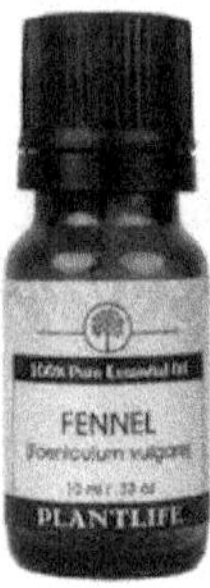

With its origins in the Mediterranean, the Fennel plant from which this essential oil is extracted from has been used as a special herb and spice in everything from food to medicine. This oil can boost both your energy and your metabolism just by breathing in its aroma. Greatly aiding in digestion, a good dose of fennel oil can greatly improve all of your metabolic processes.

Hawthorn Oil

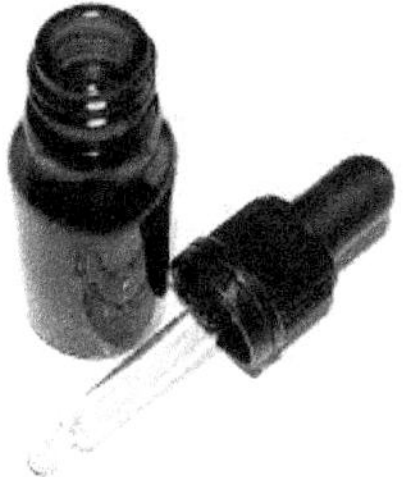

Hawthorn oil is able to strengthen the heart as it energizes the rest of the body. This essential oil serves to give your metabolism a reset, making it stronger than ever. It does this through special proactive properties that help circulate blood flow and revitalize basic bodily function giving a major boost to energy and metabolism. In order to give yourself the boost you need this winter, try a steady dose of hawthorn oil!

Peppermint Oil

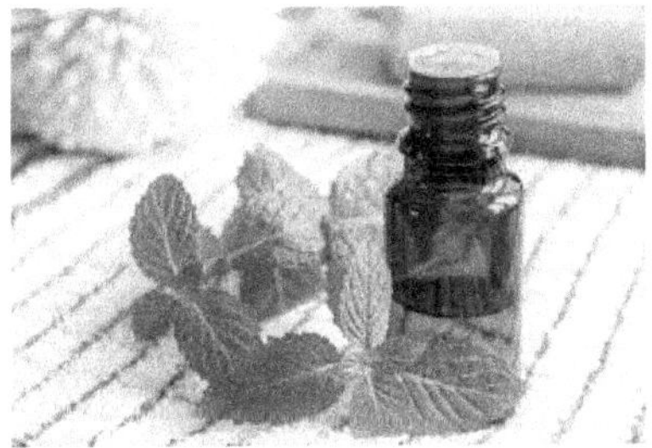

Peppermint is a common fixture during the winter months. It's on our candy canes and it resides on our peppermint patties, but believe it or not, the use of peppermint oil goes even farther back in the annals history than last Christmas! Peppermint oil has been used in India for thousands of years; referred to as "pudina ka tel" peppermint is used in Ayurvedic medicine as a powerful cleansing agent for the skin.

It utilizes several valuable vitamins and minerals such as Omega 3 fatty acids, calcium, iron, calcium, Vitamins C and A, and potassium. All of these vitamins and minerals come together to give you some of the best energy you could have during the winter season. Peppermint works to combat metabolic problems such as bloating and gas, while speeding up the rate of your metabolism in general.

Gurmar Oil

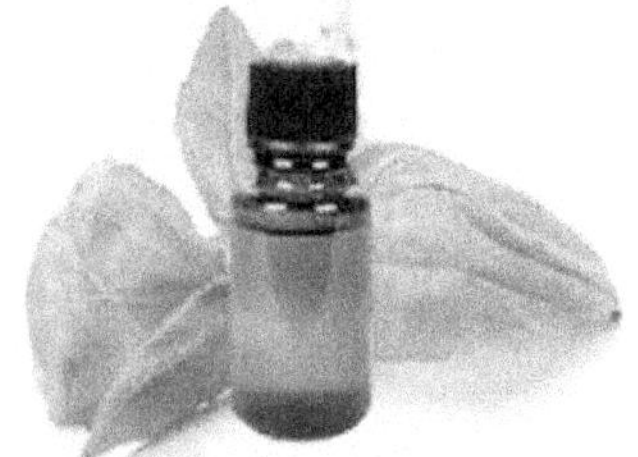

This amazing oil can help to redirect metabolic cravings such as a desire for sweets and other harmful food additives. Gurmar can help regulate blood sugar and it refines the metabolic activity of the liver, kidneys, and spleen. It also helps promote the health of your pancreas which serves to boost the overall efficiency of metabolism. If you want to keep your weight down and feel more energetic during the winter, be sure to give gurmar essential oil a try.

Seaweed Oil

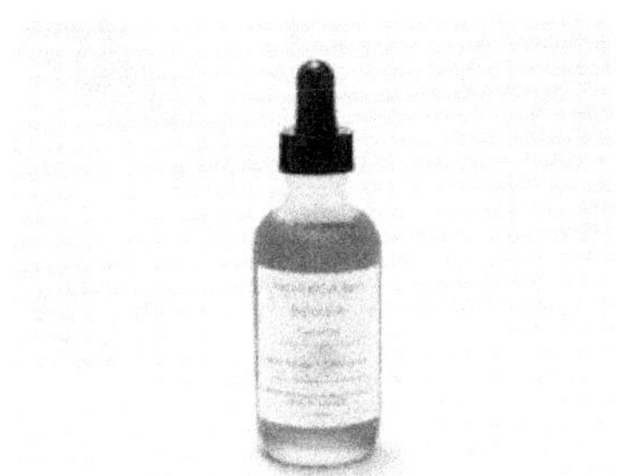

Yes, oil extracted from seaweed can do quite a bit for your metabolism, especially during the winter months. The compound called "Fucoxanthin", the element that gives seaweed its greenish brown pigmentation, has proven metabolism boosting capabilities. It is this compound along with the healthy dose of iodine that this oil contains, that contributes to a higher energy level and metabolism for those who use it. So if you are feeling more tired than you should be during the winter months, give this seaweed essential oil a try.

Prickly Pear Oil

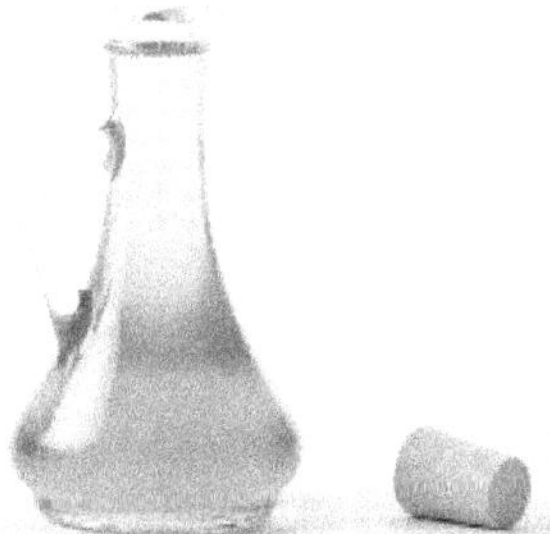

The plant from which this essential oil is derived, hails from the Cactaceae family and is quite commonly found in Mexico, the United States, and South America. It's easy to spot with its big leaves, long stems, and oval shaped pads. These prickly pairs are absolutely loaded with vitamins and minerals such as riboflavin, niacin, vitamin-B6, and thiamin. Regular doses of these vitamins and minerals will serve you well when it comes to balancing out hormone and energy levels leading to good metabolism.

Along with being such a good metabolic aid, prickly pear oil also helps our brains release serotonin, bumping up our melatonin levels allowing us to have a more restive sleep during the night, and more energy during the day. The best way to administer this oil is to dilute it with a good carrier oil base, and rub the mixture directly into the skin. You can also add this oil to your bathwater making for a great rejuvenating effect during the winter.

Conclusion: It's cold outside!

The winter weather can really take a toll on us; both mind and body can be affected by the sudden drop in temperature and decrease in sunlight. We are products of our environment, and when our environment becomes frozen and deteriorates, without proper preventative measures we might find that we begin to deteriorate as well. This book has sought to find some of the best essential oil solutions to some of the most common wintertime problems. I hope that the lessons in this guide serve you well, so that you can have the utmost of health and well being even when it's unbearably cold outside! Thank you for reading!

FREE Bonus Reminder

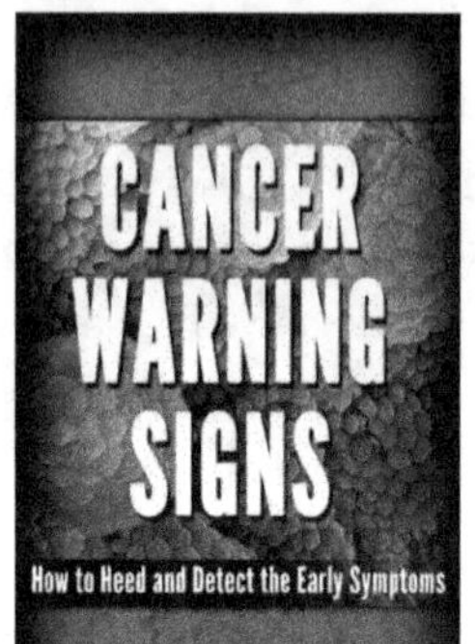

If you have not grabbed it yet, please go ahead and download your special bonus report *"Cancer Warning Signs. How To Heed & Detect The Early Symptoms!"*
Simply Click the Button Below

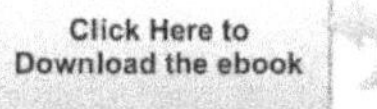

OR **Go to This Page**
http://healthylivingpeople.com/free/

BONUS #2: More Free & Discounted Books or Products

Do you want to receive more Free/Discounted Books or Products?
We have a mailing list where we send out our new Books or Products when they go free or with a discount on Amazon. Click on the link below to sign up for Free & Discount Book & Product Promotions.
=> **Sign Up for Free & Discount Book & Product Promotions** <=

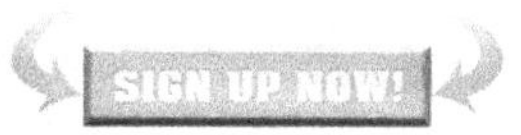

OR Go to this URL
http://zbit.ly/1WBb1Ek